Intermittent Fasting 101

How to Heal the Body, Lose Fat and Boost Energy

© Copyright 2020 - All rights reserved.
The contents of this book may not be reproduced, duplicated or transmitted without direct written permission from the author.
Under no circumstances will any legal responsibility or blame be held against the publisher for any reparation, damages, or monetary loss due to the information herein, either directly or indirectly.

Legal Notice:
You cannot amend, distribute, sell, use, quote or paraphrase any part or the content within this book without the consent of the author.

Disclaimer Notice:
Please note the information contained within this document is for educational and entertainment purposes only. No warranties of any kind are expressed or implied. Readers acknowledge that the author is not engaging in the rendering of legal, financial, medical or professional advice. Please consult a licensed professional before attempting any techniques outlined in this book.

By reading this document, the reader agrees that under no circumstances are is the author responsible for any losses, direct or indirect, which are incurred as a result of the use of information contained within this document, including, but not limited to, —errors, omissions, or inaccuracies.

CONTENTS

Introduction 1

Chapter One: What is Intermittent Fasting? 3

Chapter Two: Why Choose Intermittent Fasting? 7

Chapter Three: The Stages of Intermittent Fasting 11

Chapter Four: The Benefits of Intermittent Fasting 19

Chapter Five: Types of Intermittent Fasting 29

Chapter Six: What to Eat and What to Avoid ... 35

Chapter Seven: Who is Intermittent Fasting For? 45

Chapter Eight: Precautions 49

Conclusion 55

References 57

Introduction

The human body is incredible and can stay optimally functioning if you take care of it, but most people neglect their health until they see signs of disease. One of the most common health issues that people around the world face is excessive weight gain. The modern-day diet is filled with processed foods that are non-nutritious and do more harm than good. You need to understand that food is meant to replenish your body with essential nutrients that will help it function well. This is why it is important to eat the right food.

An unhealthy diet is where most health issues start for the majority of people. Thankfully, people have become more conscious about their health in recent years. They realize the negative impact of excess weight and an unhealthy body, but this realization also pushes them to try a lot of different fad diets. If you have tried different diets but have not found success, you know what we are talking about. But you're in luck! Here you will learn about a diet that works and will help your body in more ways than one. Intermittent fasting will help you burn all that unwanted fat, heal your body, and boost energy levels like never before.

Being overweight has a negative impact on your physical as well as mental health. Things get worse when you try unhealthy diets that show no results. Even if you count every single calorie you consume, or if you have only soup for a month, it doesn't guarantee weight loss, but fasting is an age-old method of losing weight and staying healthy. While intermittent fasting has only started gaining popularity in recent years again, the concept has existed for many years. This doesn't mean that you have to starve yourself for days at a time. It just involves short periods of fasting, followed by periods of healthy eating.

As you read the book, you will learn more about intermittent fasting in detail. The point is, this diet is a healthy practice that you can inculcate in your daily routine in many ways. It won't leave you stressing over exactly what you are eating or how many calories every bite contains. Instead, you will learn more about what food your body needs to live well and how much of it. Once you try intermittent fasting, you will see your body transform and feel the positive difference it makes in your life.

Chapter One: What is Intermittent Fasting?

Before we begin, it is important to understand that intermittent fasting is not a diet; it is an eating pattern. During intermittent fasting, you have to alternate between periods of fasting and eating.

There is no restriction about what foods you should eat or how much, but you need to exercise basic self-control with your portions when you want to lose weight. You can't expect weight loss when you fast for a whole day and eat twice the amount of junk food the next day. Not only will this make you gain more weight, but it will also do more harm than good to your body.

Eating the right food that will offer nourishment to your body is always an important aspect of good health. You can still enjoy a little of your favorite snacks once in a while, but try not to consume more than necessary, but this is something you have to decide for yourself. Intermittent fasting will help you lose weight regardless of what you eat, as long as you follow the eating pattern recommended.

Intermittent fasting can be done in many ways. In the next section, you will learn more about the different types of intermittent fasting in detail. The common factor in them is that your day or week will be split into fasting and eating periods.

Fasting is already something that most people do every day. The whole time you are sleeping, your body is fasting. In intermittent fasting, you just have to increase those fasting hours a little. The most common and effective method of losing weight through intermittent fasting is by following the 16/8 rule. Here you will be fasting for 16 hours and eating your meals within 8 hours. By restricting your eating window, you automatically reduce the number of calories you consume in a day. During fasting hours, your body turns towards the stored fat in your body for energy instead of the food you eat.

You might think that intermittent fasting is too difficult, but in reality, it is fairly easy. Adjusting to this new eating pattern will require a little self-discipline at first, but you soon get used to it. Intermittent fasting is not about starving yourself for days on end. Instead, you just fast for short periods and thus promote the process of fat burning. Most people find that their energy levels are boosted after they get used to intermittent fasting in their daily routines. This eating pattern will also help you feel better than you usually do.

The constant consumption of unhealthy processed or junk food does more harm to your mind and body than you realize. Such food will constantly cause hunger pangs and cravings and lead to mood swings. By eating better and restricting your eating time, your body can heal and return to its healthy state again.

Hunger may be an issue at first, especially for those who constantly tend to eat something throughout the day, but once you stick to intermittent fasting for a while, your body gets the chance to get accustomed to it. You won't feel as hungry as usual, and your body gets used to not consuming food all the time.

During the fasting period, you should only have water or beverages that have no calories. This could be tea or coffee but without any sugar, milk, etc. Staying hydrated is an important part of fasting healthily. People also take health supplements during the fasting period, but these should be non-calorific too. There are also types of intermittent fasting that allow you to consume small amounts of low calorific food instead of going completely calorie-free. This depends on the health conditions, lifestyle, and personal choices made by people.

So now you understand what intermittent fasting

involves. As you read on, you will learn more about how it works and how to start intermittent fasting.

Chapter Two: Why Choose Intermittent Fasting?

A lot of people assume that fasting is the same as starvation, and starvation is a bad thing, so why should we fast? But fasting is not the same as starvation. When you fast, you voluntarily stop yourself from eating. When you starve, it is an involuntary act where your body has no access to any food. While the latter is dangerous, the former does a lot of good for the body.

Fasting has been a time-tested tradition in many parts of the world. Not only does fasting help you lose weight, but it also extends life, improves concentration, improves insulin resistance, and has other benefits.

When it comes to weight loss, people focus too much on what they should eat. The forgotten aspect of weight loss is when one should eat. Understanding the importance of eating at the right time is just as important as learning about the right food for your body.

When you eat food, it increases the insulin levels in the body. Regardless of what you eat, there will always be an increase in insulin levels after eating. When you eat healthy food, there will be a normal increase in insulin levels. When you eat the wrong foods, there is an unhealthy high in insulin levels. But the key takeaway is that eating increases insulin secretion. If you want to prevent insulin resistance in the body, you periodically have to let the body sustain itself on a very low level of insulin. So fasting or the voluntary restriction of eating is the only answer.

Fasting is tried and tested as compared to other fad diets out there. Don't expect miracles from exotic new diets. Instead, use this ancient method that people have benefited from for many years. Nearly every culture or religion in the world mentions fasting. While people fast for a few hours, others can last for days. But here, you will learn about the benefits of intermittent fasting, where you alternate between eating and fasting.

Hippocrates, the father of modern medicine, was also in favor of fasting. Plato, Aristotle, and Plutarch echoed these sentiments as well. You will see a mention of many supporters of fasting throughout history.

History of Intermittent Fasting

In ancient medicine, it was believed that nature was the best healer. When a person or an animal becomes sick, they don't eat. Think back to the last time you fell sick; you will notice that appetite is drastically reduced during such times. Fasting is an instinct that is present in all of us during illness. According to the ancient Greeks, fasting can improve the cognitive abilities of a person. Think back to the last time you had a big meal during the holidays. Did you feel lazy and sleepy or energetic and alert after the meal? The answer is more likely to be the former.

When you eat too much, more blood is directed to your digestive system to deal with the huge amount of food intake. This means that there is less blood flow to the brain, and it causes a somewhat dopey feeling. So when you do the opposite of eating too much, the results will also be the detrimental. Intermittent fasting will not make you weak and lazy. Instead, it will increase blood flow to the brain and help you become more energetic and alert.

It was not just the Greeks that supported the practice of fasting. The founder of toxicology, Philip Paracelsus, as well as Benjamin Franklin, were in favor of fasting. They believed that fasting was better than any other medicine and helped the body heal faster.

Fasting is also prominent in spiritual practices, and nearly every major religion believes it supports the practice of fasting. In spiritual terms, fasting is said to be an act of purification or cleansing. But if you look at it scientifically, it still means the same thing. By fasting, you give your body the chance to get rid of toxins and any harmful substances. While the practice itself may be conducted in different ways, it has the same principle.

As you can see, the idea of fasting has been present for a very long time. If it were truly a harmful practice, we would have figured it out by now. Fasting has withstood the test of time purely because it is beneficial for the human body and should be a part of our routine.

Chapter Three: The Stages of Intermittent Fasting

As mentioned before, intermittent fasting isn't a miracle solution to weight loss. It won't help you shed 10 pounds in a week or give you any such results that other fad diets may promise. At its best, intermittent fasting is a lifestyle transformation that will do you a world of good. It helps your body become a lot more efficient and boosts your immunity as well.

During the process of intermittent fasting, there is a lot that happens. These things don't happen at all when you eat a lot, or else they take place at a very slow rate, but you need to induce such processes in your body to lose weight and to regain good health.

Five Stages of Intermittent Fasting

- Ketosis

- Autophagy

- Growth hormone

- Insulin reduction

- Immune cell rejuvenation

When your body is in a well-fed state, the cells in the body are in growth mode. The insulin signaling and the mTOR pathways will tell your cells to grow, divide, and synthesize proteins. If these pathways are overactive, they have serious implications in the growth of cancer cells.

The mTOR is the mammalian target of rapamycin. It likes having a lot of nutrients like proteins and carbohydrates around. If it is active, it tells the cells in your body not to conduct autophagy. Autophagy is a process where the cells cleanse themselves and get rid of any damaged proteins. When your cells are well fed, they don't care about being efficient and conducting autophagy. Instead, they focus more on dividing and growing.

Cells and their components are very acetylated when they are in a well-fed state. This means that the molecules in the cells have acetyl groups attached to their lysine residue. This jargon may not make sense to you right now, so don't pay much heed to it. You need to understand that the many genes in your well-fed cells are turned on, including those that are important for proliferation and survival on a cellular level. The acetylation causes the packaging proteins to loosen up, and protein production easily takes place with the DNA being read.

When you are in this well-fed state, genes are turned on while others are turned off. The ones that are turned off include genes that are linked to stress resistance, fat metabolism, and damage repair. Your stored fat gets converted to ketone bodies during fasting, and these reactivate these important genes. This then lowers inflammation and allows better resistance to stress in the brain.

Things are different when you starve. While fasting, the body sees the low availability of food as environmental stress and then changes the expression of genes that protect you from stress. There is a starvation program in the body that kicks cells into a very different mode when there is no glucose available at all.

During fasting and exercising, the AMPK signaling pathway is activated. AMPK acts as a brake for mTOR. It will signal your cells to go into a self-preservation mode during autophagy and fat metabolism activation. MTOR is inhibited. NAD+ molecules rise during fasting as well since there aren't enough sugars or proteins that usually allow the conversion of these molecules to NADH in the Krebs cycle. Instead, these molecules will activate sirtuins called SIRT1 and SIRT3. Resveratrol in wine helps promote a long life because it can potentially activate sirtuins in the body too. This helps you understand the significance of sirtuin activation. Sirtuins are proteins that can remove the acetyl groups from proteins like histones.

During fasting, ketones are produced, and these keep acetyl groups in place or function as deacetylate inhibitors. It turns on the genes that are linked to damage repair and antioxidant processes.

As you can see, fasting allows a lot of things to happen in your body. It can undo most of the damage that is caused by overeating and constantly keeping the body in an over-fed state.

In about 12 hours of fasting, ketosis kicks in. During ketosis, the body will start breaking down the fat cells that are stored in the body and burn them for energy. The liver uses the fat to produce ketone bodies. Ketones or ketone bodies are an alternative source of energy in the body. A lot of people assume that glucose is the only way to keep the body energized the body, but can also burn fats for energy. When you constantly eat food, you provide the body with an endless supply of glucose. This is why it is unable to use the stored fat for energy. Instead, eating too much means you are taking in more glucose than you need, and this extra food gets stored as fat as well.

Ketones serve as an energy source for your brain, heart, and skeletal muscle when there is a lack of sufficient glucose in the body. When your body is resting, the brain uses nearly 60 percent of the glucose for energy. During fasting, your body gets the opportunity to use ketones as fuel for the brain and other organs. Because of this usage of ketone bodies by the brain, you will experience better mental clarity and stable moods. Glucose produces a lot more inflammatory products during metabolization than ketones do. Ketones can also stimulate the production of BDNF, which is the brain growth factor. Studies have shown that ketones reduce the amount of cell death or cell damage in neurons while reducing inflammation in other types of cells.

After 18 hours of fasting, the body goes into an active fat-burning mode and generates a lot more ketones. At this point, it is possible to measure the levels of blood ketones. Normally, blood ketone levels fall between 0.05 and 0.1 mmol/l, but fasting or carbohydrate restriction increases the concentration between 5-7 mmol/l.

As ketone levels in the bloodstream increase, they work similarly to hormones and act as signaling molecules. Ketones tell the body to boost any pathways that will reduce inflammation and repair any damaged DNA.

If you fast for 24 hours, your cells will keep recycling the old components within them and break down any damaged proteins. Such misfolded proteins are usually linked to conditions like Alzheimer's disease. The process that takes place here is autophagy.

Autophagy is a very important process in the body since it allows the rejuvenation of cells and tissues. This process helps remove misfolded proteins and any other cellular components that are damaged. When your cells fail to initiate autophagy, it can lead to the onset of neurodegenerative diseases. These diseases tend to develop when there is reduced autophagy in the body with increased age. Autophagy is activated when fasting stimulates the AMPK pathway while inhibiting mTOR activity.

This will only happen when the glucose stores in your body are substantially depleted, and insulin levels start dropping. In studies conducted on mice, it was seen that autophagy increases significantly after 24 hours of fasting. This process's effect is even more prominent in brain and liver cells when you fast for 48 hours. In studies conducted on humans, autophagy was detected in neutrophils after a person fasts for 24 hours. Autophagy is further increased in the body when a person exercises while fasting.

After 48 hours of fasting, the body's growth hormone level can increase fivefold compared to when you just began fasting. The ketones produced while fasting stimulates the secretion of growth hormone. The hunger hormone Ghrelin is also a promoter of growth hormone secretion. The growth hormone allows the preservation of muscle mass in the body and reduces the accumulation of fat tissue. These things tend to occur increasingly as we age. This is why it is important to fast and counter this effect of aging. Intermittent fasting has been known to promote mammalian longevity. It promotes better cardiovascular health and faster wound healing.

After 54 hours, insulin levels drop to the lowest point since the onset of fasting. This allows the body to become a lot more insulin sensitive. There are many health benefits associated with lower insulin levels. Lowering the levels of insulin in your body will help you see the long-term as well as short-term benefits. It will stop the insulin and mTOR signaling pathways while activating autophagy. It will also help reduce inflammation, make you more insulin sensitive, and protect you from diseases usually linked to aging.

Within 72 hours of fasting, the body starts breaking down any old immune cells and generates new ones. This is seen in prolonged fasting more than intermittent fasting. Fasting for this long will cause reduced circulation of IGF-1 levels and lowers PKA activity. Insulin-like growth factor 1 is similar to insulin and promotes growth in most cells in your body. It also activates the PI3K-Akt pathway and other signaling pathways that promote cell growth and survival. Prolonged fasting can lead to better stress resistance and allow cell regeneration and renewal. It has also shown a positive effect on the preservation of white blood cells in patients who undergo chemotherapy.

The last stage of intermittent fasting is not fasting but re-feeding. Since your aim is not to kick the body into starvation mode, you have to break the fast at some point. Having a nutritious and balanced meal after fasting will help to promote better cell functions. In the re-feeding stage, insulin sensitivity is improved, and there is better stress resistance as well as cognition. Your meal should have a balanced amount of carbohydrates, fats, and proteins. Avoid consuming too much sugar or carbohydrates. Carbohydrates fill you up but don't help your body much. A little of it is more than enough for your energy supply. Avoiding processed foods and simple sugars will help your health in the long run.

Now you understand a lot more about what happens in the body when you try intermittent fasting. It is up to you to fast for 10 hours, 16 hours, or even 48 hours if you can. As you make progress in your journey with intermittent fasting, you will watch as all the things mentioned here are manifested in your body.

Chapter Four: The Benefits of Intermittent Fasting

Many studies have shown that intermittent fasting has powerful benefits for the mind and body. Intermittent fasting can bring about positive metabolic changes on a cellular level. It can initiate the natural secretion of hormones such as insulin and human growth hormones that are essential for the body's physical development. There are a lot more benefits you will reap from it. Learning about these benefits will further convince you to give this eating pattern a try for yourself.

Health Benefits of Intermittent Fasting

Improves Function of Genes, Cells, and Hormones

A lot of different things happen in the human body

when you don't eat food for a while. Certain cellular repair processes are initiated, and the hormone levels change as well so that your body can access the stored fat for energy. The following are the changes that occur when you fast:

Insulin Level

The blood level of insulin will see a significant drop when you fast. This will help the process of burning fat.

Human Growth Hormone

The levels of growth hormone in the blood can see a 5 fold increase during fasting. The higher the level of the growth hormone, the more fat is burned. There is also a lot of muscle gain, along with other benefits.

Cellular Repair

Intermittent fasting can induce cellular repair processes that are important for the body. For instance, it promotes the removal of any waste material from the cells.

Gene Repair

Certain changes take place in genes and the molecules that are linked to immunity and longevity.

Weight Loss

It can help you burn belly fat and lose weight. This is one of the prominent reasons why most people try intermittent fasting. While weight gain happens almost unconsciously fast, losing weight is a struggle for most people, but intermittent fasting can help you lose weight quite fast. You will be eating fewer meals than usual and thus be taking in fewer calories. It is important not to overeat during the non-fasting period, or the entire purpose is defeated. Other than the reduced intake of calories, weight loss is also facilitated by the changes in hormone levels caused by fasting.

The high levels of growth hormone, low levels of insulin, and increased secretion of norepinephrine will help the breakdown of stored fat. This will allow the body to use fat for energy instead of glucose. Short term fasting can increase the metabolic rate in the body anywhere between 3 to 15 percent. This means that you will be burning a lot more calories than you usually do.

Not only does intermittent fasting help you consume a lower amount of calories, but it also increases the number of calories that are burned. A study conducted by Patterson R. et al. (2015) inferred that people who try intermittent fasting could lose at least 3-8 percent of their excess weight within a period of 3 to 24 weeks. This may seem less, but is actually a significant amount of weight loss. Along with the overall weight loss, there is a 4-7 percent reduction in their waist circumference. This is especially important since most people struggle with losing abdominal fat. Having too much-stored fat in the abdominal cavity can lead to serious illness.

The study also showed that intermittent fasting would cause very little muscle loss compared to continuous calorie restriction. Instead, it can lead to muscle gain. The more muscle in the body, the more fat is burned.

All in all, intermittent fasting is a powerful tool for weight loss.

Help Control Diabetes

It can reduce insulin resistance and lower the risk of Type 2 diabetes. In recent years, Type 2 diabetes has become increasingly common. This condition's main feature is that blood sugar levels are extremely high, with insulin resistance. So when insulin resistance is reduced, blood sugar levels reduce as well. This means that you can be protected from the risk of developing Type 2 diabetes. Interestingly, many studies have shown that intermittent fasting reduces insulin resistance and reduces blood sugar levels.

According to studies, a person on intermittent fasting can reduce their fasting blood sugar level by anywhere between 3-6 percent while their fasting insulin reduces by about 30 percent. Since intermittent fasting promotes the regulation of insulin production in the body, it is significant in managing symptoms related to Type 2 diabetes. Another study conducted by Tikoo K. et al. (2007) on diabetic rats showed that intermittent fasting helped in protecting them from kidney damage. This was an important inference since kidney damage is a severe complication associated with diabetes, but results may differ with respect to genders and may also depend on the individual.

Helps Reduces Oxidative Stress and Inflammation

Oxidative stress has a strong impact on aging and can also cause other chronic illnesses. Free radicals react with protein, DNA, and other important molecules and cause damage. These free radicals are unstable molecules. With intermittent fasting, there is increased resistance in the body to oxidative stress. It can also fight inflammation, which can lead to or be a symptom of other diseases. Intermittent fasting can significantly lower the body's oxidative stress. This means that the level of toxins and free radicals in your body will reduce if you often practice intermittent fasting.

Good For Your Heart

Heart disease is one of the most common fatal diseases around the world. More people die from heart conditions than most other diseases. There are many risk factors that are linked with a higher or lower risk of heart issues. Intermittent fasting can help to reduce the risk of many such factors. It can help to support healthy blood pressure, cholesterol, triglyceride, and blood sugar levels. While these have only been proven scientifically on experiments done in animals, a lot of people have experienced similar results after intermittent fasting. Intermittent fasting requires you to restrict your calorie intake. You will be receiving your nutritional requirements through healthy and balanced meals. This proves to be very beneficial for cardiovascular health. Since intermittent fasting can reduce the body's cholesterol levels as well as blood pressure, this is very good for the heart and the circulatory system. A lot more studies still need to be conducted to justify that intermittent fasting can be recommended by medical professionals to achieve these benefits.

Cellular Repair

Fasting initiates a process called autophagy in the body. Autophagy is a waste removal process that takes place in cells. It involves the breakdown of cells along with the metabolization of dysfunctional and broken proteins within the cells. These proteins usually build up in the cells over long periods. When more autophagy takes place, it helps to protect the body against various illnesses such as Alzheimer's disease and cancer. Intermittent fasting promotes recovery and repair of the body's cells. Proper nutrition allows the cells to perform metabolic activities. This significantly helps in the healing and regeneration of cells and tackling general inflammation.

Can Help Prevent Cancer

When a person has cancer, there seems to be an

uncontrolled growth of cells in their body. According to research conducted by de Groot S. et al. (2019), fasting may have beneficial effects on the metabolism of a person and thus reduce their risk of developing cancer. While more scientific proof is required to ascertain this, studies have shown that intermittent fasting reduces the side effects that cancer patients suffer from during chemotherapy.

Good For The Brain

Things that are good for the human body are usually good for the brain too. Intermittent fasting has a beneficial effect on certain metabolic functions that also promote good brain function. It helps to reduce oxidative stress, blood sugar levels, insulin resistance, and blood sugar levels. Studies conducted on rats have also suggested that intermittent fasting may help promote the growth of nerve cells and thus promote brain function. These studies have also shown that intermittent fasting protects against brain damage that is often caused by a stroke. What is healthy for the body is also healthy for the brain. A reduction in oxidative stress and blood pressure can significantly improve brain health and neural functions. Intermittent fasting has shown positive results and an increase in the growth of nerve cells in studies conducted on animals.

Helps Prevent the Onset of Alzheimer's Disease

Alzheimer's disease is a neurodegenerative disease

that is quite common around the world. To date, there is no known cure for this illness. This is why it is critical to try to prevent its onset in the first place. A study conducted by Halagappa, V. K., et al. (2007) on rats showed that intermittent fasting might be helpful in this. It may help reduce the severity of the condition when it develops or help prevent the disease.

Another study named 'Reversal of cognitive decline: A novel therapeutic program' carried out by Bredesen D (2014) stated that 9 out of 10 Alzheimer's patients demonstrated an improvement in their symptoms when they included intermittent fasting into their daily routine. Other studies suggest that intermittent fasting may help protect against other neurodegenerative conditions, like Huntington's disease or Parkinson's disease.

Longevity

Intermittent Fasting can help you live a longer life. Other than weight loss, this may be one of the more enticing benefits of intermittent fasting. Short periods of fasting may help to extend our lifespan. According to studies on rats, intermittent fasting works similar to calorie restriction in extending the expected lifespan. A few of these studies have very dramatic results as compared to others.

A study conducted by Goodrick, C. L., et al. (1982) showed that rats that fasted every other day would have 83 percent more lifespan than those that did not fast. Such research has made intermittent fasting a popular topic of discussion in forums about anti-aging. A lot of people have included such short-term fasts into their routine in an attempt to increase longevity. The most important benefit of intermittent fasting is an increase in the longevity of an individual. Since intermittent fasting brings about positive changes from the cellular levels, it can significantly reduce your chances of contracting diseases. This means that you get to live a longer and healthier life.

Chapter Five: Types of Intermittent Fasting

Intermittent fasting does not have to be done in a particular way. There are quite a few different types of intermittent fasting that you can try.

Six Popular Methods That You May Try for Yourself

16/8 Method

This is one of the most common and effective methods of intermittent fasting. It involves a daily fasting period of 14-16 hours with an eating period of 8-10 hours. Within the eating period, you can choose to have two or three meals. People choose to have smaller portions at frequent intervals instead of three big meals during the eating window. This 16/8 method was popularized by Martin Berkhan, a fitness expert, and is also called the Lean Gains protocol. If you want to think of this method simply, just focus on not having any food after dinner and skipping breakfast. For instance, you can fast for 16 hours if you have dinner at 8 p.m. and lunch at noon the next day without eating anything in between. According to experts, women should opt for a 14-hour fast instead of 16 hours. This shorter fasting period seems to work better for them. If you usually skip breakfast, this is an easy method of eating to inculcate into your routine, but someone who gets very hungry in the morning can find it difficult to skip breakfast initially. You can curb hunger pangs during the fasting period by drinking water, tea, coffee, and any calorie-free beverages. Eating healthy foods within the eating period is important if you want to lose weight and improve your health. If you end up eating a lot of junk food after the fasting period, it will not help you see any positive results at all. Instead, you may end up gaining more weight.

5:2 Method

In this method of intermittent fasting, you will be allowed to eat as you usually do on 5 days of the week, but your calorie intake should not cross 600 on the other two days of the week. This method is known as the Fast diet, and it was made popular by Michael Mosley, a British journalist. On this diet, women are recommended a limit of 500 calories on the two fasting days, and men can have about 600 calories. If you follow this method, set a schedule for yourself. For instance, if you want to restrict calorie intake on Mondays and Fridays, every other day can involve normal meals, but on these two days, count your calories and try sticking to two small meals. While there aren't specific studies that confirm the benefits of this method, intermittent fasting itself is beneficial in any form.

Eat Stop Eat Method

In this method, you have to fast for 24 hours once or twice a week. Fitness expert Brad Pilon was responsible for popularizing this particular method. You can complete a 24-hour fast by avoiding any meals after dinner the previous day until dinner the next day. For instance, if you have dinner at 8 p.m. on Tuesday, you can only eat your next meal at 8 p.m. on Wednesday. The period in between will be the 24 hours fast. You can switch it up according to your preference. You need to fast between breakfast one day and breakfast the next day or between lunches if you prefer. The result will be the same as long as you complete 24 hours of fasting. Solid foods are not permitted while fasting, but you can have any zero-calorie beverages like water or black coffee. To be able to lose weight effectively, eat healthy normal meals on other days. Don't try to compensate for your fasting period by eating more within the eating window. The downside of the eat stop eat method is that most people find it difficult to fast for a full 24-hour period. If you can start with a complete 24-hour fast, you can start by fasting for 14 hours, then 16, and slowly building your way to 24 hours.

Alternate Day Fasting Method

As the name suggests, alternate-day fasting requires you to fast on alternate days. This method has a few different versions. These allow you to consume 500-600 calories, even on the fasting days. Beginners may find it difficult to complete a whole day of fasting every alternate day, so it is not usually recommended to them. If you choose this method, you have to be prepared for going to bed hungry half of the days in the week. This type of intermittent fasting should not be followed in the long term and is better suited for a short period. It is unsustainable and difficult for people to follow.

Warrior Diet Method

You may have heard of this method that was popularized by Ori Hofmekler, a fitness expert. The warrior diet involves the consumption of one big meal for dinner and small portions of raw vegetables and fruits for the rest of the day. It means that you can feast at night after fasting the whole day. The eating period at night is only 4 hours. This method is one of the popular intermittent fasting models followed by people around the world. The food recommended on this diet is similar to the food choices for those following the Paleo diet. You need to avoid processed foods as much as possible and instead opt for wholesome, nutritious food.

Spontaneous Meal Skipping Method

There is no structured plan for this type of intermittent fasting. You can reap its benefits by simply skipping meals when you can. People don't need to consume food every few hours. You won't lose muscle or enter starvation mode by skipping a meal or two. In fact, the human body is capable of withstanding days without food, so a missed meal will do you no harm. On days that you don't feel very hungry, don't force yourself to eat much. It is okay to skip lunch if you are too busy. When you skip a meal, just make sure that your next meal is a healthy one. A short fast will help your body and allow you to reap the benefits of intermittent fasting.

Intermittent fasting will work differently for different people. While one method may be very easy for someone to follow, another person may find it extremely difficult. This is why it is helpful that there are so many types of intermittent fasting methods for people to try. You can choose the one that you feel will be simpler for you to follow. Choosing a method that is too difficult for you will only cause you to give up on intermittent fasting even before you see any benefits from it.

Chapter Six: What to Eat and What to Avoid

As you already know by now, intermittent fasting is more about the when than what or how much, but paying attention to what you eat is a very important aspect of losing weight and gaining a healthy body. It is essential to apply certain fundamental nutrition principles to your practice of intermittent fasting, regardless of which method you follow.

What you eat is even more important when you try intermittent fasting since you will be undergoing long periods without food. This means that you should try your best to provide your body with healthy food during the eating period between fasting.

Intermittent fasting does not specifically mention any restrictions on what or how much food to eat, but if you accompany the process with a big cheeseburger during your eating period, you will not see any positive results.

What To Eat

Before you adopt any stringent diet plans, always make sure that you consult a health professional to make sure that it is the best decision for your body type. Although the term "fasting" seems very ominous and difficult, "intermittent fasting" is something that has caught a lot of traction in the already crowded world of dieting and fasting.

Several studies suggest that following the intermittent fasting regime can lead to significant weight loss and stabilize blood sugar levels. This is a big reason behind the growing popularity of intermittent fasting.

The biggest appeal of intermittent fasting is the lack of stringent rules; there are restrictions on what you eat but not many limitations on what one can eat, but this does not mean that gorging on junk food during the feeding window is going to do you any favors. Downing, a whole bag of potato chips or a tub of ice cream in between fasts, is probably not the right way to go. That is why we will be looking into the best foods to include in your Intermittent Fasting diet.

Most experts suggest that a well-balanced diet is a

key to losing fat and maintaining good energy levels while on a stringent intermittent fasting diet. Anyone who has adopted the intermittent fasting diet plan should focus on eating nutrient-rich foods like whole grains, vegetables, fruits, seeds, beans, lean proteins, and dairy products. It is important to note that these dietary recommendations are normally suggested for improving one's health, even if not for intermittent fasting.

Water

Technically, water may not be considered food, but biologically, it is considered the most important nutritional requirement for any human being. Water is important for the general well-being of any major organs of the body. You would be very surprised if you have been thinking of surviving your fast without considering water as a part of it. The amount of water that every person requires on a daily basis varies depending on height, weight, gender, climate conditions, and physical activity levels. The best measure to detect a shortage of water (dehydration) is urine color. Urine should appear pale yellow at all times if one is healthy. A darker shade of yellow suggests that you are dehydrated. Other symptoms of dehydration are fatigue, headaches, light-headedness, and a lack of energy. If dehydration is accompanied by limited food intake or consumption of unhealthy food, you have got yourself a recipe for disaster. If the idea of drinking plain water does not excite you, you can make things more flavorful by adding a squeeze of lemon juice or mint leaves and cucumber slices in your water.

Avocados

Although eating fruit with the highest calorie count may seem counterproductive to one's quest of losing weight, avocados are one of the best things that you can incorporate into your diet while following intermittent fasting. Due to their high content of unsaturated fat, avocados will help you to feel full even during the most intense periods of fasting.

Research studies have confirmed that unsaturated fats will help the body to keep full and maintain energy levels even if you don't feel full. The human body is capable of giving off signs to show that it has enough nourishment inherently to prevent it from going into starvation mode. Unsaturated fats are capable of prolonging these signs for longer periods of time, even if you might be feeling a little hungry while you are in the middle of a fasting period. A recent dietary study conducted by Wien, M., et al. (2013) finds that even adding half an avocado in your lunch will help you stay full for a longer time.

Seafood and Fish

There is a reason why most dietary guidelines or meal plans suggest eating three or four-ounce servings of fish every week. Seafood and fish contain ample amounts of vitamin D, in addition to being extremely rich in proteins and healthy fats. Since intermittent fasting predicates you to eat during limited time periods, you will need more nutritional food intake during these limited time windows, and chowing on seafood and fish is the best way to make sure that. Additionally, there are lots of ways to cook fish and seafood, which means that you will never run out of foods to create tasty dishes.

Cruciferous Vegetables

Vegetables such as cauliflower, broccoli, Brussels sprouts, and other cruciferous greens are high in fiber content. When you are only eating food during certain intervals of the day, it is crucial to make sure that your diet includes fiber-rich foods that will help you support digestive health and help your poop factory run smoothly. Fiber-rich foods such as cruciferous vegetables will also help you to stay full, which is always an advantage when you are not eating for 16 hours a day. The consumption of cruciferous vegetables will also help you to reduce the risk of developing cancer and other health problems.

Potatoes

Not all carbohydrate-rich foods are bad. A research study that was conducted by Akilen, R., et al. (2016) found that potatoes are one of the most satiating foods. The study says that incorporating potatoes into your diet can help with weight loss and loss of body fat, but the way you eat potatoes also makes a huge difference; gorging on fried potato chips or French fries won't help your cause.

Beans and Legumes

Beans and legumes can be your best friend while following the Intermittent Fasting lifestyle. Foods containing a high content of carbs are the main energy source for biological activities. Carbo-loading with a ridiculous amount of food is not what you should do, but it will not hurt you if you throw in low-calorie carbohydrates such as legumes and beans in your diet plan. These foods will help your body to stay perked-up even during peak fasting hours. Chickpeas, lentils, peas, and black beans have been found to decrease body weight even without the presence of a calorie restriction or calorie deficit.

Probiotics

The little critters and bacteria that are a part of your gut biome love diversity and consistency. This means that your gut biome can get depleted when you are hungry or fasting. When your gut biome is not at its best, it can manifest itself through irritating side effects such as constipation and other digestive problems. To be able to deal with these unpleasant effects, adding foods that are rich in probiotics can do the trick. Sauerkrauts, kombucha, kefir, and curd are rich in good bacteria and aid the gut biome in functioning well.

Berries

If you are a big fan of smoothies and healthy shakes, berries are a great choice. Berries are loaded with vital nutrients, and that is not even the best part about it. A research study conducted in 2016 found that people who regularly consume berries with lots of flavonoids such as strawberries and blueberries observed smaller changes in BMI over the long run when compared to people who did not consume berries.

Eggs

Eggs are loaded with proteins and vitamins; a single egg contains up to 6.5 grams of proteins and a plethora of vitamins. Getting as much protein as possible is extremely important when it comes to building muscle mass and maintaining enough energy levels in your body, especially when you are eating within a limited period of the day. In other words, it is a convenient and healthy solution if you want to eat something during an 8-hour feeding window.

Nuts and Dried Fruits

Although dried fruits and nuts may contain many calories compared to other snacks, they contain something that most snack foods don't - good fats. If you are worried about consuming too many calories, keep your mind at peace. It has been discovered that a single ounce of almonds contains 20 percent fewer calories than what is listed on the label or packaging. Another important bit of information that makes a case for nuts and dried fruits stronger is that chewing the nuts does not completely break down the product's cell walls. This means that most of it stays intact, and the body does not completely absorb it while digesting it. If you eat almonds every day, they might not affect your daily calorie intake as much as one would like you to believe.

Whole Grains

Eating carbs while on a restrictive diet plan may seem counterproductive to your weight loss aspirations, but you will be very relieved to know that this is not always the case. Unprocessed whole grains provide a lot of proteins and fibers, which means that eating a decent serving of it goes a long way to help you keep full and maintain energy levels. The healthiest whole grains that can be incorporated into your diet while following an intermittent fasting plan are amaranth, farro, bulgur, spelled, kamut, freekeh, sorghum, and millets. Whole wheat is also a good choice as long as it is consumed in controlled portions.

What Not To Eat

When it comes to avoiding certain types of food, the choices are very clear, and one should basically avoid junk food and highly processed food products. Foods that have been prepackaged and last for a long time are loaded with additives and preservatives that can affect your body more severely while on an intermittent fasting plan. Basic food products that you will need to avoid are:

- Fast Foods

- Sweetened Fruit Juices

- Sweets

- Sugary Sodas

- Processed Foods (including processed grains).

- Complex carbohydrates.

Chapter Seven: Who is Intermittent Fasting For?

Intermittent fasting has been associated with a number of health benefits. The process puts your body in a state of starvation and induces the burning of stored fats to provide energy.

Who Should Try Intermittent Fasting?

Intermittent fasting is especially beneficial for people who want to lose weight or reduce body fat percentage.

Intermittent fasting is also effective for people who are suffering from appetite disorders. Depriving the body of food for a period can induce hunger. People who are recovering from chemotherapy or hypertension have a lowered food intake capacity. Intermittent fasting can help stimulate the appetite of such individuals.

In short, intermittent fast is beneficial for the body if you do not suffer from any pre-existing medical conditions. People who are eating unhealthy or living unhealthy lifestyles can reshape their health and fitness by switching to intermittent fasting instead of a conventional diet.

Who Should Avoid Intermittent Fasting?

Intermittent fasting may not be dangerous, but it is not meant for everyone. Intermittent fasting is not for you if you have higher caloric requirements. You may feel tired, hungry, dehydrated, and irritable. Intermittent fasting is not easy to follow, which means even if you are healthy, don't have an eating disorder, are over 18 years of age, aren't pregnant, or breastfeeding, you will still have a few side effects.

Intermittent fasting can sometimes lead to dehydration. A lot of people forget to drink water while fasting. Hydration is important, or you will feel tired, as the body will be running in less energy than usual. Fasting can also boost stress levels, which can also disrupt sleeping patterns. Your stomach may grumble during your fasting periods. Avoid smelling or looking or thoughts related to food as it can discharge gastric acids in your stomach. Non-fasting days are the days when you can eat anything you want, but this may lead to weight loss. Fasting can lead to a spike in your stress hormones, such as cortisol, which can lead to more cravings.

The biggest side effects of intermittent fasting are binge eating and overeating. The biochemistry that controls your mood also controls your appetite, which affects the actions of neurotransmitters like serotonin and dopamine, which may lead to depression and anxiety. It means that the deregulation of your appetite has the same effect on your mood, which may lead to you feeling irate on occasions on the day you are fasting.

People who have diabetes are on anti-diabetic prescriptions, such as insulin. Anti-diabetic medications have an effect on your blood sugar while you're fasting. This drops the sugar levels extremely low. People who are diabetic should maintain steady blood sugar, but intermittent fasting doesn't allow that. If you want to train for a marathon, intermittent fasting is not for you.

Timely nutrition is important for endurance sports, so it is advisable not to fast if you are into sports. Sports requires a lot of calories because it burns a lot of calories. Endurance exercise requires consistent calorie intake and adequate macronutrient intake to repair muscles, replenish glycogen, and support electrolyte balance. So intermittent fasting cannot offer a steady dose of nutrients and calories that are needed to exercise, perform, and recover.

Chapter Eight: Precautions

Intermittent fasting is a popular eating pattern. It involves not eating or restricting your food intake for a certain period. This fasting method has been linked to many potential health benefits, changes in gene expression, and a short-term increase in human growth hormone, but it can be dangerous if not done properly. Here are precautions to help you fast safely.

Keeping Fasting Periods Short

There isn't just one single way to fast. That means the duration of your fasting period is up to you. Most of the regimens include short fasting periods of 8-24 hours. People undertake longer fasts of 48 and even up to 72 hours. Longer fasting periods can increase your risk of side effects, including irritability, mood changes, lack of energy, hunger, fainting, dehydration, and inability to focus. The best way to avoid the side effects is by sticking to shorter fasting periods up to 24 hours.

Stay Hydrated

Dehydration causes fatigue, headaches, and dry mouth, so you should drink enough fluid while fasting. While you get 20-30 percent of the fluid from food, you can easily dehydrate while you are on a fast. To prevent dehydration, you should listen to your body and drink when thirsty.

Eat Small Amounts on Fast Days

As you can remove food altogether, fasting patterns allow you to consume up to 25 percent of your calorie requirements in a day. It may make fasting sustainable, since you likely won't feel hungry. It may also reduce many of the risks associated with it, such as feeling faint and unfocused. You can restrict your calories and still eat small amounts that may be a safer choice than doing a full-blown fast.

Don't Break Fasts With a Feast

It can be tempting to eat a huge meal after a period of restriction. Breaking a fast with a feast could make you feel bloated and tired. Feasting may also harm your long-term goals by halting your weight loss. Try easing gently back into your regular eating routine.

Go for Walks or Meditate

To avoid eating on fast days can be difficult. To avoid unintentionally breaking your fast is to keep yourself busy. Any activity that is not too stressful and is calming, like taking a bath, reading a book, or listening to a podcast, walking, or meditating, can keep your mind engaged.

Giving Up Too Soon

Intermittent fasting will be grueling and difficult during the first weeks. You will need to stay hungry for prolonged periods of time without eating any food or snacks. Regardless of the type of intermittent fasting you decide to practice; it requires a certain level of discipline to be able to stick to the routine. During the first few weeks, you will need to overcome your hunger pangs and be mentally strong if you want your efforts to be successful. If you are able to get through these initial difficulties, you will begin to see the positive benefits of intermittent fasting. You will have to trust the diet and make an effort to stick to it to see positive results.

Binge Eating

After your fasting period is completed, you will certainly be tempted to overeat to satisfy your hunger, but overloading on calories after fasting for 16 hours will negate the positive effects of the diet. After a period of prolonged fasting, overeating will do you no good and cause your weight to increase, so you need to resist the desire to overeat and pace yourself to control your food intake. The stomach realizes that it is full only after 20 minutes from when you eat your meals, so taking your time and eating slowly is the correct way to go about intermittent fasting.

Not Eating Enough

You will need to eat the proper amount of food and not eat too little or too much. If you do not eat properly after breaking your fast, your body will stay in a state of starvation. This will prevent you from achieving your weight loss goals and health goals. It is common for people to believe that they will undo the positive effects of fasting and avoid eating properly after breaking a fast, but it will make it more difficult for you to get through the next fasting period if you do this. Your body needs food to be able to function optimally. Skipping meals or not eating enough will only be counter beneficial and will do you no good.

Eating the Wrong Foods

You will need to eat the right food to reap all the benefits that intermittent fasting provides for the body. The quality of the calories that you consume is as important as the number of calories you consume. For instance, your 16 hour fast will be completely useless if you eat a tub of ice cream right after. You need to take care of what you eat as your body processes different types of calories in different ways. For instance, 500 calories derived from avocados will be metabolized differently as compared to 500 calories derived from ice cream. Junk food is always bad for health so avoid eating it after fasting. A healthy and balanced diet is an important part of the intermittent fasting diet. Make sure that you consume all the macronutrients before you decide to eat any junk food after fasting. You need to fill yourself with food that is rich in proteins, fibers, healthy fatty acids, and carbohydrates before deciding to chew on a chocolate bar.

Taking it Too Far

People tend to think that more is better. The advisable fasting period does not exceed 16 hours, but people feel that a longer fast translates to more weight loss, and they push themselves to fast for longer periods. This has no positive effect, and you need to know when to stop, but you also need to make sure that you don't develop a habit of breaking your fast too early.

Conclusion

By now, you know a lot about intermittent fasting. Learning about the diet instead of following it blindly will help you understand why it will work instead of leaving you stranded like other fad diets. Intermittent fasting is fairly simple and easy for most people to follow. Not only will it help you lose weight, but it also has a lot of other benefits that you can reap in the long run.

It teaches you to eat better instead of consuming a lot of unhealthy processed food. You also learn to listen to your body instead of constantly consuming more than the body needs. Fasting for short periods gives your body the chance to use all the calories you consume and also burn through the stored fat. You might find it a little difficult to fast for long periods at first, but it only takes a while to get used to this new dietary plan.

Once you start seeing the results, you will be even more motivated to follow through with it. Make intermittent fasting a part of your daily life and watch it heal and improve your body. You will soon find yourself recommending this diet and maybe this book to friends and family as well.

References

Akilen, R., Deljoomanesh, N., Hunschede, S., Smith, C. E., Arshad, M. U., Kubant, R., & Anderson, G. H. (2016). The effects of potatoes and other carbohydrate side dishes are consumed with meat on food intake, glycemia, and satiety response in children. Nutrition & diabetes, 6(2), e195. https://doi.org/10.1038/nutd.2016.1

Bredesen, D. (2014). Reversal of cognitive decline: a novel therapeutic program. In Aging. Retrieved from Buck Institute for Research on Aging website: https://www.aging-us.com/article/100690

Fung, D. J. (2015, April 11). Fasting - A History. The Fasting Method website: https://thefastingmethod.com/fasting-a-history-part-i/

Goodrick, C. L., Ingram, D. K., Reynolds, M. A., Freeman, J. R., & Cider, N. L. (1982). Effects of intermittent feeding upon growth and life span in rats. Gerontology, 28(4), 233–241. https://doi.org/10.1159/000212538

de Groot, S., Pijl, H., van der Hoeven, J., & Kroep, J. R. (2019). Effects of short-term fasting on cancer treatment. Journal of experimental & clinical cancer research: CR, 38(1), 209. https://doi.org/10.1186/s13046-019-1189-9

Gunnar, K. (2016, August 16). 10 Evidence-Based Health Benefits of Intermittent Fasting. Healthlinc website: https://www.healthline.com/nutrition/10-health-benefits-of-intermittent-fasting#TOC_TITLE_HDR_11

Gunnars, K. (2017, June 4). What Is Intermittent Fasting? Explained in Human Terms. Healthline website: https://www.healthline.com/nutrition/what-is-intermittent-fasting#TOC_TITLE_HDR_3

Halagappa, V. K., Guo, Z., Pearson, M., Matsuoka, Y., Cutler, R. G., Laferla, F. M., & Mattson, M. P. (2007). Intermittent fasting and caloric restriction ameliorate age-related behavioral deficits in the triple-transgenic mouse model of Alzheimer's disease. Neurobiology of disease, 26(1), 212–220. https://doi.org/10.1016/j.nbd.2006.12.019

Jarreau, P. (2019, February 26). The 5 Stages of Intermittent Fasting. LIFE Apps | LIVE and LEARN website: https://lifeapps.io/fasting/the-5-stages-of-intermittent-fasting/

Patterson, R. E., Laughlin, G. A., LaCroix, A. Z., Hartman, S. J., Natarajan, L., Senger, C. M., Martínez, M. E., Villaseñor, A., Sears, D. D., Marinac, C. R., & Gallo, L. C. (2015). Intermittent Fasting and Human Metabolic Health. Journal of the Academy of Nutrition and Dietetics, 115(8), 1203–1212. https://doi.org/10.1016/j.jand.2015.02.018

Tikoo, K., Tripathi, D. N., Kabra, D. G., Sharma, V., & Gaikwad, A. B. (2007). Intermittent fasting prevents the progression of type I diabetic nephropathy in rats and changes the expression of Sir2 and p53. FEBS letters, 581(5), 1071–1078. https://doi.org/10.1016/j.febslet.2007.02.006

Wien, M., Haddad, E., Oda, K., & Sabaté, J. (2013). A randomized 3×3 crossover study to evaluate the effect of Hass avocado intake on post-ingestive satiety, glucose and insulin levels, and subsequent energy intake in overweight adults. Nutrition journal, 12, 155. https://doi.org/10.1186/1475-2891-12-155

Printed in Great Britain
by Amazon